Hangov

Solved

Robert Walker

Published by LifeBodyEnergy™ Publishing.

Contact email, rob@hangoverssolved.com

Hangovers Solved, www.hangoverssolved.com

The book contains my opinions on how the body functions. The contents of the book have been formulated through my own experiences. The views expressed are my theories and have not been verified, evaluated or approved by anyone from a scientific or medical organisation or background. I do not recommend that anyone ceases taking any medication, or changes their medical treatment unless instructed to by their doctor. This book has been written strictly for informational purposes only. It is not intended to provide medical advice or to be any form of medical treatment. Any use of the information in this book is the reader's decision, and is solely the reader's responsibility. I do not advocate excessive drinking of alcohol; I am always mindful of recommended levels of alcohol consumption and drink responsibly.

ISBN: 9781973239314

Cover Design: www.spiffingcovers.com Tel 01206 585 200 email: enquiries@spiffingcovers.com

Table of Contents

ONE

Hangovers Solved Overview

Taking sufficient vitamin C POWDER after drinking alcohol before you go to sleep MAY help prevent you suffering from a hangover, or improve on how you usually feel after consuming alcohol.

The process described in this book worked for me and others.

There is no guarantee it will work for you since your body's workings are unique to you.

This book is not a miracle cure and it will require some effort to achieve results.

My website, www.hangoverssolved.com contains the most up-to-date information.

My contact on Twitter is @HangoversSOLVED.

TWO

Introduction

After drinking alcohol, I discovered that taking sufficient vitamin C POWDER mixed with water BEFORE going to bed, meant that I woke up without a hangover.

The effort which you need to put in involves you following a simple process to determine how much vitamin C POWDER your body requires after drinking alcohol, in order to prevent you waking up with a hangover, or an improvement on how you currently wake up feeling after drinking alcohol.

Your body is unique to you and only you can identify the amount of vitamin C POWDER it requires to help prevent a hangover. Once you have established this, it is simple to calculate how much vitamin C POWDER you need to take after consuming a small, medium or large amount of alcohol. If you do not put in a small amount of effort to calculate your body's vitamin C requirements, and you rely on a trial and error approach, you may find you have to run to the loo, experience diarrhoea and still wake up with a hangover.

I found that this process only worked for me if I used vitamin C in POWDER form and mixed it with water.

Please drink responsibly at all times. Alcohol is a double-edged sword; it can help provide enjoyment, but it can also cause huge problems for you, your health and wider society as a whole.

Do you drink alcohol because you want to or because you feel you need to?

If you drink because you feel you need to, then you need to question if you are self-medicating with alcohol to help deal with pressures and stress in your life. This may not damage your health too much in the short-term, however, it is not advisable to drink heavily in the longer term, and remember there are never any answers to be found at the bottom of a bottle.

THREE

What Causes Hangovers?

The key factor is that you consume more alcohol than your body is able to process.

The book provides advice on how taking sufficient vitamin C POWDER before you go to sleep could assist your body's ability to process alcohol.

The time you go to bed may also have bearing on how you feel after drinking alcohol. I believe that the body completes certain housekeeping functions between the hours of 23.00 and 04.00, as part of its daily rhythm. If you drink alcohol beyond 23.00, not only are you impairing the body's housekeeping routine, you are also presenting your body with an additional huge task to complete in processing the alcohol you have consumed. These additional burdens may help to explain the lethargy some people feel the day after drinking alcohol.

If you stay up until the early hours of the morning, even if you do not consume alcohol, you will find your body feels out of sync the next day, and so the importance of trying to go to bed as early as possible should be borne in mind.

It may be prudent to bring your alcohol consumption forward to earlier in the day in order for you to finish drinking earlier in the evening, however, this may not always be feasible. If you are able to stop drinking by 21.30, take some vitamin C POWDER and eat some food, this may allow you to be in bed by 23.30, which I believe will help process any alcohol consumed more efficiently.

FOUR

Why Drink Alcohol?

It is important to be able to answer this question honestly, at least to yourself.

Alcohol tastes good to most people and they also like the effects it has on them.

Do you drink because you want to or because you feel you need to?

Alcohol is probably one of the most popular stress relievers; after a few sips, all can seem well with the world again. Do you drink as a response to stress in your life?

There are other responses to choose to help manage stress. You could listen to your favourite music, go for a walk or take a nap. These responses do not place a burden on your body like alcohol does, they help you naturally.

The best response to stress is to identify the root cause and to solve it to prevent stress reoccurring. This will probably take much more effort on your part, but positive actions that reduce stress are worth the investment of your time and energy.

Do you drink alcohol because of habit? Have you always done this? Are you addicted to drinking alcohol? Try stopping for one month to prove to yourself that you can.

Do you drink because of peer pressure? Other people may be self-medicating with alcohol and are simply looking for a drinking buddy.

Alcohol can be very enjoyable and make for some really fun times, but respect alcohol, respect your body and please drink responsibly.

FIVE

Alcohol Warning

If you drink a large amount of alcohol and take some vitamin C POWDER before you go to sleep as this book suggests, you may wake up without a hangover like I do.

You may feel fine, with no headache or nausea and think about going about your normal daily business, however, your body will still be under the influence of alcohol and you should not drive a vehicle or operate machinery.

When you wake up you should drink some tea, coffee, juice or water, eat some breakfast and remain mindful of whether you feel your body and mind is in any way impaired.

Do not take any chances that may endanger yourself or risk the lives of other people. Sadly, some people are killed every week as a result of drink-driving, please be sensible and help to eradicate these unnecessary fatalities.

Damage Caused By Hangovers

If you are suffering with a hangover your body is in a state of distress, and your ability to function physically, mentally and emotionally is severely impaired. If you take vitamin C POWDER before you go to sleep to help prevent damage to your health, then this is a positive action.

There are days off work taken due to people suffering hangovers which will affect workplace productivity.

A person suffering a hangover may waste a whole day or even longer incapacitated in bed simply recovering from a few drinks.

Children will suffer from poor parenting if the parent is hungover.

Doctors and hospitals have to waste huge amounts of resources in dealing with people that have consumed more alcohol than their bodies are able to process.

Your health and well-being is precious and has limits to the damage it can endure, so please treat your body with the respect it deserves.

Please drink responsibly and do not use the protection that vitamin C powder may provide you with, as an excuse to drink dangerous quantities of alcohol.

SEVEN

Solving Your Hangovers

The concept is very simple; you drink alcohol, you mix vitamin C POWDER with water, take before you go to sleep and wake up hangover free, or at least feeling better than you usually do after consuming alcohol.

The above process worked for me and others and it may work for you, however, your body's internal chemistry is unique to you, and there are no guarantees.

The only item which you need to purchase is vitamin C POWDER, and links to the Amazon UK and Amazon USA vitamin C store listings can be found on my website www.hangoverssolved.com

Please take time when making your purchase and ensure you buy vitamin C in POWDER form; I found the hangover prevention process only works for me when I use vitamin C POWDER.

Firstly, you need to calculate the quantity of vitamin C POWDER your unique body requires, to help prevent suffering from a hangover.

The recommended daily amount advised to be taken in most countries is 1 or 2 grams. I found through my testing that if I had drunk a large volume of alcohol, approximately 10 (Great British) pints or 5.5 litres (5,500ml), then my body required 50 grams of vitamin C POWDER. This quantity of vitamin C could cause severe diarrhoea for some people, hence the requirement for you to individually calculate the quantity your body requires. I am unsure if there is any relationship between a person's physical attributes and their vitamin C requirements, but for your information, I am approximately 1.9m (6'3"), 95kg (15 stone/ 210lbs) and have a large frame. I was 32 years old when I first calculated my vitamin C needs.

I have read extensively about vitamin C; there is a wealth of information online detailing the benefits which humans may derive by consuming vitamin C supplements daily. There are articles which explain how taking vitamin C 'mega-doses' can assist human health.

The first time I took a 50g dose of vitamin C to prevent a hangover was in 2005. I do not take vitamin C on a daily basis since I eat a diet rich in vitamin C-containing fruits and vegetables.

EIGHT

Calculating Vitamin C Quantity to Take

I found vitamin C powder to be the key vitamin that prevented me from suffering with a hangover. I had read extensively about the various health benefits that vitamin C can supposedly provide the body with.

An article suggested taking one teaspoon of vitamin C powder (5g) every thirty minutes until you need to run to the loo and experience a watery stool. The article claimed that this exercise will provide you with your body's vitamin C tolerance level.

Once you have determined what your unique vitamin C tolerance level is, this figure can be used as a basis for calculating how much vitamin C you need to take to prevent suffering with a hangover. This is the process I designed and it has never failed to work for me.

In order for you to complete this test, you need to purchase some vitamin C powder. I completed the exercise while I was at home on a day off from work, and I also had the following day off too. I had not drunk any alcohol the previous day.

It is important to be near to a toilet that you have quick unimpeded access to, since when you feel you need to go to the toilet you will need to go very quickly.

I suggest that you also purchase some moist toilet tissue wipes. It is likely that you will have several visits to the toilet over a few hours, and using only standard toilet paper may leave you with a sore bottom.

I ate my normal breakfast and waited for one hour until it had settled before I started taking vitamin C.

I used my digital kitchen scales to weigh out 5g of vitamin C powder. I put the powder into a mug and I covered with lukewarm water from the kettle, since I found this dissolved the powder most effectively. I only used approximately 100ml of water to dissolve the vitamin C powder; the smaller the amount of water you use, the easier it is to consume quickly.

The taste is extremely bitter and the mixture is very acidic and so not good for your teeth. You may need to have a small sip of juice or smoothie to take away the bitter taste in your mouth. I would recommend that you minimise the amount of juice, since you do not want it to compromise the accuracy of the test.

After you have consumed your dose of vitamin C mixture and maybe juice as well if required, it is very important to immediately rinse your mouth out five times with plain water, to help clean any acidic residues from your teeth. Do not brush your teeth since you may inadvertently brush the acid in your mouth into your teeth and gums.

Repeat the above process every thirty minutes until you experience a watery stool. Write the time down on a piece of paper after each dose so you stay on schedule. Set your alarm or use an accurate kitchen timer to prompt you to take the next dose of vitamin C.

When I completed the exercise it took ten hours, and I consumed 100g of vitamin C until I had to run to the toilet.

I did not eat or drink anything during the process. My stomach felt full and made various gurgling noises throughout the day, and I felt a gradual build-up of pressure which ended when I had to run to the toilet.

When I did experience a watery stool, it was a fairly explosive episode so please stay as near to a toilet as is feasible for you. It would also be prudent to wear loose-fitting and easy to adjust clothes, since when you feel you need to go to the toilet, you will need to go quickly.

Once you have experienced a watery stool do not take any further vitamin C, simply record the total weight of vitamin C powder that you have taken. It is likely that you will feel loose for several hours and possibly even into the following day. I suggest wearing several layers of underwear in bed and the next day until you feel like your body has returned to normal functioning. You should expect several subsequent trips to the toilet, although none should be as explosive as the initial watery stool visit.

When you have completed the above exercise, you will have identified your body's unique vitamin C tolerance level. The level may be as low as 10g or as high as 100g like it was for me. You will be using this information to help calculate the optimum amount of vitamin C to take to help prevent you suffering from a hangover.

I found through the above process that my vitamin C tolerance level was 100g. I used this information as a base to experiment taking varying amounts of vitamin C powder after I had drunk alcohol, to test whether it prevented me from waking up with a hangover.

The optimum amount of vitamin C powder for you to take to prevent suffering with a hangover will depend primarily on the quantity and strength of alcohol that you have consumed.

The figures below are the quantities of how much vitamin C I found prevented me from getting a hangover. As previously stated, your body is unique in the world and you will need to ascertain the quantities which work for you.

If I consumed a large amount of alcohol, i.e. 10 GB Pints/ 5.5 Litres lager / 1.5 Litres Wine then I took 50% of my vitamin C tolerance level. My vitamin C tolerance level was 100g multiplied by 50%; I therefore took 50g vitamin C powder (10 teaspoons).

If I had consumed a medium amount of alcohol, i.e. 7 GB Pints /4 Litres lager / 1 Litre Wine then I took 33% of my vitamin C tolerance level. The calculation therefore was 100g multiplied by 33%; I therefore took 33g vitamin C powder (6.5 teaspoons).

If I had consumed a small amount of alcohol, i.e. 4 GB Pints/ 2 Litres lager / 0.5 Litre Wine then I took 20% of my vitamin C tolerance level. The amount therefore was 100g multiplied by 20%; I therefore took 20g vitamin C powder (4 teaspoons).

If you are not managing to prevent suffering with a hangover after consuming alcohol by following the above process, please read the chapter, 'It Is Not Working.'

NINE

Taking Vitamin C

Your body and its internal chemistry is unique to you, therefore only you can calculate and determine the quantity of vitamin C powder to take before going to bed, to hopefully prevent you waking up with a hangover.

You will need to use the results of the exercise in the previous chapter, as a guideline to determining the vitamin C dosage you require, which will also be based upon how much alcohol you have drunk, and what strength the alcohol was.

The maximum amount of vitamin C powder that I could comfortably consume in a drink was 20g dissolved in a mug, any amount greater than this tasted too bitter for me. If I had drunk a large amount of alcohol, I knew from previous experiences that I needed to take 50g of vitamin C powder. In order for me to be able to drink the 50g of vitamin C powder, I mixed two mugs of 20g each with water, and one mug of 10g. Please note that I always used my digital kitchen scales to accurately weigh the amount of vitamin C powder.

Whenever I drank large amounts of vitamin C powder as described above, I immediately sipped some sweet smoothie to help take away the extremely bitter taste. I also rinsed my mouth out with water five times to try to help minimise any damage to my teeth.

If you feel that you will struggle to mix vitamin C powder with water when you get home after consuming alcohol, you could prepare the mix in advance and store in small beakers with a lid. You could place these beakers on your stairs, at your bedside or in another location you deem suitable. You may need to give the beakers a shake, or stir the mixture when you are ready to consume them, since after several hours the vitamin C powder and the water may separate.

TEN

It Is Not Working

Most people lead busy lives and free time is at a premium. There are some people that said they did not have time to calculate their vitamin C tolerance level as explained earlier in the book. These people decided to simply adopt a trial and error method of taking vitamin C powder before going to sleep after a night drinking alcohol.

There have been mixed results with adopting this short-cut method.

Some people found taking one teaspoon of vitamin C powder after consuming a small amount of alcohol, two teaspoons after consuming a medium amount and three teaspoons after a large amount, prevented them waking up with a hangover or improved on how they used to feel after drinking.

Other people found that the trial and error approach resulted in them experiencing diarrhoea and still waking up with a hangover. If this is your experience then I can only suggest that you follow the vitamin C tolerance exercise to see if it provides you with better results.

I can only tell you what worked for me, which is completing the vitamin C tolerance test prior to using vitamin C powder as prevention from suffering a hangover.

The notes below are my opinions about the body and what may assist you in being able to prevent suffering from hangovers.

I researched about hangovers, the body and specifically the liver. I concluded that vitamin C is to the liver, what fuel is to a vehicle, i.e. if you run out of fuel, you are going nowhere, and if your liver exhausts its vitamin C stores you will suffer with a hangover.

When your liver runs out of vitamin C, alcohol will continue to circulate in your body and cause untold damage. The greater the amounts of unprocessed alcohol flowing around your system, the more acute your hangover symptoms are likely to be.

It is likely that you will continue to feel ill, until you have consumed some food and drink which contains vitamin C. The progress to feeling better will be slow since your body has a backlog of alcohol processing to be completed, hence why some people say they suffer with a three day hangover.

Why do some people take vitamin C after consuming alcohol and suffer with diarrhoea and still wake up with a hangover?

I believe this is because the vitamin C does not complete its journey to the liver, it finds itself being side-tracked with another task on en-route.

The digestive tract stretches from the mouth to the bottom. It is possible that a person's digestive tract may be obstructed with pockets of food residues and debris. If a person consumes a vitamin C mixture to try to prevent a hangover, this mixture could react with and wash away the debris, thus causing the diarrhoea and using up the vitamin C for this task, rather than the job of preventing a hangover which it was designated for.

Please appreciate that this theory of mine is just a theory based upon my own personal research and experience.

So what options do you have if you are seemingly unable to prevent hangovers?

The first recommendation is that you complete the vitamin C tolerance test. This will completely clean out your system and potentially mean that any future vitamin C taken, may complete its journey to the liver and help prevent a hangover.

Please note that I completed several of these vitamin C tolerance tests, which some people refer to as vitamin C flushes. I completed them since I had read that keeping the body's vitamin C levels topped up can help improve our health in general. I completed these flushes at the rate of one per month, since it really is a 'belt-and-braces' way to clear out the digestive tract, and a recovery period is desirable.

There are many ways to clean out the digestive tract without completing a vitamin C flush. The juicing of green cabbage produces an astringent liquid which may clean out your insides, it certainly did for me. A diet that involves eating a whole lettuce and whole cooked cabbage everyday will also act as a cleanser for the digestive tract.

The purpose of cleaning out the digestive tract is that vitamin C taken to prevent a hangover, does actually complete its route to the liver. How a person chooses to clean out their digestive tract is their choice.

I undertook a program of a few vitamin C flushes, many weeks of juicing sweetheart cabbages daily, and also eating lots of green vegetables. The results of this regime cleaned out my insides and also contributed to me losing weight. When I took the vitamin C mixture to prevent a hangover at a later date, it did not result in me suffering with diarrhoea, and I woke up feeling fine.

ELEVEN

Hints and Tips

There are a number of measures you can take to assist your body in lessening the effects of any alcohol consumed.

The consumption of a substantial meal prior to drinking alcohol may mean the alcohol is absorbed at a slower rate and hence its effects are not as acute.

The consumption of food after you have finished drinking may help to lessen the effects of the alcohol that you are experiencing. The cravings for types of food you experience after drinking alcohol are unique to you, and it is important to listen to what your body is telling you it needs.

It is my opinion that the liver in our bodies is like an internal pharmacy store; when we consume alcohol our body raids the liver for nutrients to help make the alcohol safe and ready for excretion. The most important nutrient I believe in this process is vitamin C which this book majors on, however, nutrients of any kind can only assist your body. After consuming alcohol I aim to drink some sweet smoothie, eat some carbohydrates such as chips/fries with salt on them, and also if available, consume some meat or fish. I also sometimes crave cheese and crackers too. It is always a good idea to sit upright for one hour to let your food digest and settle, in order to gain the optimum nutritional benefit from it.

After a night drinking alcohol, if all you feel like doing is going to sleep, then I would suggest as a minimum to take some vitamin C powder mixed with water. In my opinion this is the highest value activity you can undertake to help prevent a hangover when you wake up.

Dehydration can leave a person with a headache, even when no alcohol has been consumed. It is important to try and replace lost fluids with some water before you go to sleep, and keeping some water by your bedside to sip on in the night is also a good idea.

The time you go to bed is almost as important as how much alcohol you consume. We all know how groggy we feel after a poor sleep, and getting to bed as early as possible will help your body. I believe from my research that the body performs its "housekeeping routines" between 23.00 and 04.00, and it is my experience that the body copes better if you begin drinking alcohol earlier in the day, which may allow you to stop drinking by 21.30, eat food, take some vitamin C powder and be in by bed by 23.00; this may assist in preventing a hangover. The trend in recent years for people to go out later in the evening may be more enjoyable from a social perspective, but it is to the detriment of your body's ability to process alcohol and general well-being.

If I know I am going to be drinking a large amount of alcohol I take a teaspoon of vitamin C powder (5g) before I begin drinking.

When I have started drinking alcohol I have never taken vitamin C powder in between drinks. I am unsure what effect this would have and I decided not to do this. I believe it is feasible to think that mixing alcohol and vitamin C powder in the stomach at the same time may lead to an upset stomach. As stated earlier, your body is unique to you and only you can decide what works best for your body.

TWELVE

Help, I'm Hungover!

If you have not taken any vitamin C powder after drinking alcohol and wake up feeling ill, there are a few things which you can do but you should not expect a miraculous recovery, since your body still has to process the alcohol you drank last night. I cannot stress enough how vital it is to take vitamin C powder before you go to sleep.

Your body is playing catch-up and it can feel a little like closing the stable door after the horse has bolted, however, you may be able to limit your hangover to being one day out of your life, not three.

Firstly take some vitamin C powder as outlined in this book. As suggested earlier, only you can decide what amount to take for your body's current needs.

Drink some smoothie and sip water.

Try to eat some toast with butter and marmite since this will help mop up the alcohol, give you some energy and replace lost salt. It is important to listen to your body and to give it the food which you have a taste for, however, do not get into your car to drive and pick this food up if you are still under the influence of alcohol; a hangover can be endured but death through a road traffic accident cannot. It is therefore important to eat what food you have in your house or which you can arrange to be safely delivered.

You may benefit from taking your usual pain relief.

Once any food you eat has digested, I would suggest you lie down, sleep, watch TV or do anything which you find relaxing. Your body has got a big job to do and so preserving as much energy as possible for this task is desirable.

Continue to relax, eat, drink and take more vitamin C powder if you feel it is appropriate.

THIRTEEN

Hangover Prevention Checklist
You need to purchase vitamin C in POWDER form.

My website www.hangoverssolved.com contains links to the Amazon UK and Amazon USA stores vitamin C listings. There are some shops which sell vitamin C in powder form, however, the majority near to where I live only sell vitamin C in tablet form, and I found that these did not provide the same benefits as the powder.

If you feel you will be unable to successfully weigh out vitamin C powder and make a drink after your night out, then it may be prudent to prepare your mixture in one or several beakers prior to leaving your house. Locate these beakers strategically so that you do not forget to drink the mixtures before you go to bed.

You must take the mixture before you go to sleep- this is the single most important piece of advice I can give. If you do forget to take it before you go to sleep, then consume it as soon as you realise.

If you are away from home, ensure that you have vitamin C powder in your toiletries bag so that you are never without it. It is advisable to have a supply of vitamin C powder that you leave in your toiletries bag, since if you leave the house in a rush; it is possible that you may forget to pack it.

The progression from suffering with hangovers to being able to consume alcohol and waking up fine is a great improvement. I would urge you to exercise extreme caution when waking up without a hangover, since you are still likely to be under the influence of alcohol. Please do not put your own life in danger or that of other innocent people; many drivers are still over the safe limit to drive even twelve hours after drinking alcohol. If in doubt, miss driving out.

If you have found that by following the "vitamin C protocol" which I describe in this book, that you have consumed alcohol on numerous occasions and have woken up without a hangover, do not be lulled into a false sense of security that you no longer need to take your vitamin C powder. The first time you forget to take your vitamin C powder, you will wake up with a hangover possibly more severe than you ever previously experienced.

If you are stranded away from home and you forgot to pack your vitamin C powder then try to eat fruit or drink juice before you go to sleep. Potatoes/Chips/Fries contain vitamin C and so may also help alleviate any possible hangover in the morning. There are several vitamins and preparations available to buy which contain vitamin C, and although they do not contain the quantity of vitamin C which this book suggests your body may need, anything is better than nothing in desperate times, when you do not have any vitamin C powder with you.

It is advisable to continue to consume vitamin C- containing foods until you begin to feel better if you are without your vitamin C powder. A steady supply of satsumas and oranges eaten throughout the day will top up your vitamin C levels, provide some dietary fibre and also help to quench your thirst.

FOURTEEN

Summary
Taking vitamin C powder mixed with water before you go to sleep after a night of drinking alcohol, may prevent you waking up with a hangover like it did for me. It may at least improve on how you usually feel after a night of consuming alcohol.

The method described in this book is to help you to identify the amount of vitamin C your body needs to help prevent a hangover. Your body is unique and only you can accurately calculate your body's vitamin C requirements.

This simple process worked for me and others but there is no guarantee it will work for you.

It is not a miracle cure; if you spend six hours consuming alcohol, take vitamin C powder before going to bed and then only sleep for four hours, you cannot expect to wake up feeling fully alert and ready to go about your day. The vitamin C may have prevented a headache and nausea, however, you will still be under the influence of alcohol, and you should not drive or do anything that may put your safety or that of other people in jeopardy.

Please drink responsibly at all times and consider the recommended daily drinking limits. Alcohol can provide a fun experience, but it is also the main factor in many deaths. Treat alcohol with respect and treat your body with respect.

FIFTEEN

Acknowledgements

The time we spend on this earth is short and goes incredibly fast. You owe it to yourself to pursue a personal and professional life which you enjoy.

Setting up a business in the UK or being self-employed is fairly simple once someone has explained how to do it, and ongoing support to ensure you complete all the required forms and returns is most helpful.

I highly recommend Small Business Accountants (SBA) Limited. 85-87 Saltergate, Chesterfield, Derbyshire. S40 1JS. Telephone: 01246 232 922. Website: www.sbalimited.co.uk Email: reception@sbalimited.co.uk

They provide support to individuals and businesses across the UK.

I would also like to thank Amazon for their help in setting up an account allowing me to self-publish books on the Kindle Direct publishing platform. It is said that we all have at least one book within us and Amazon can help you to facilitate this.

I have received excellent support from www.wordpress.com for help in setting up my own website. The WordPress platforms enable you to simply create and update your own website and blog.

If you need help designing a book cover, website and other digital media work I recommend SpiffingCovers, 6 Jolliffe's Court, 51-57 High Street, Wivenhoe, Colchester, Essex. CO7 9AZ. Telephone 01206 585 200. Website: www.spiffingcovers.com Email: enquiries@spiffingcovers.com

Printed in Great Britain
by Amazon